Table Of Contents

Introduction

Welcome to the world of holistic health, where wellness is understood as more than just the absence of disease. Holistic health embodies a comprehensive approach to well-being, acknowledging the intricate interplay between the mind, body, and spirit. This introduction will explore the foundational concepts, historical roots, and modern applications of holistic health, offering insights into how you can embrace a more balanced and fulfilling life.

Holistic health is grounded in the belief that health is a dynamic state of being, achieved through the harmony of physical, emotional, mental, and spiritual dimensions. Unlike conventional medicine, which often focuses on treating specific symptoms or diseases, holistic health seeks to address the underlying causes of illness and promote overall well-being.

At its core, holistic health recognizes that the body is an integrated whole, where every part is interconnected. It emphasizes the importance of lifestyle choices, environmental factors, and emotional states in influencing health. By considering the full spectrum of an individual's life and experiences, holistic health aims to cultivate a state of balance and harmony.

The origins of holistic health can be traced back to ancient civilizations that practiced medicine in ways that honored the whole person. Traditional Chinese Medicine (TCM), for instance, has been practiced for over 2,000 years, emphasizing the balance of the body's vital energy, or Qi, through acupuncture, herbal remedies, and physical exercises like tai chi.

In India, Ayurveda, one of the world's oldest holistic healing systems, has been practiced for over 3,000 years. It focuses on balancing the body's energies through diet, herbal treatments, and yogic practices, tailored to an individual's unique constitution and life circumstances.

Native American healing traditions also play a significant role in the history of holistic health. These practices emphasize the connection between humans and nature, utilizing rituals, herbal medicine, and spiritual ceremonies to promote healing and balance.

In the Western world, the principles of holistic health can be found in the teachings of Hippocrates, the "Father of Medicine." Hippocrates emphasized the healing power of nature and the importance of diet and lifestyle in maintaining health, laying the foundation for holistic approaches in modern medicine.

Today, holistic health has evolved to integrate both ancient wisdom and contemporary scientific knowledge. It encompasses a wide range of practices and therapies, including:

Integrative Medicine: Combining conventional medical treatments with alternative therapies such as acupuncture, massage, and nutritional counseling.

Functional Medicine: Focusing on identifying and addressing the root causes of disease through personalized treatment plans.

Mind-Body Medicine: Utilizing techniques like meditation, yoga, and biofeedback to enhance the mind's influence on physical health.

Natural Therapies: Emphasizing the use of natural remedies, such as herbal medicine and nutrition, to support the body's innate healing processes.

Holistic health also promotes preventive care and wellness, encouraging individuals to adopt

healthy lifestyle habits, manage stress effectively, and engage in regular physical activity. By

fostering a holistic perspective, people can achieve a greater sense of balance and fulfillment in

their lives.

As you embark on your journey into holistic health, it's important to remember that this approach

is about more than just treating illnesses; it's about creating a lifestyle that supports your overall

well-being. Whether through dietary changes, mindfulness practices, or exploring new forms of

therapy, holistic health offers a path to a more balanced, vibrant, and harmonious life.

In the pages that follow, we will delve deeper into the various dimensions of holistic health,

providing practical guidance and insights to help you integrate these principles into your daily

life. Embrace the journey towards holistic well-being and discover the transformative power of

caring for the whole person.

What Is Holistic Health?

In today's fast-paced world, the quest for health and wellness has led many to explore holistic health, an approach that considers the entire person rather than just addressing symptoms or specific ailments. Holistic health emphasizes the interconnection between mind, body, and spirit, aiming to achieve a harmonious balance that fosters overall well-being. This chapter delves into the essence of holistic health, its defining principles, and the multifaceted ways it enhances our lives.

Holistic health is an approach to wellness that considers the whole person, including their physical, mental, emotional, and spiritual dimensions. This philosophy is rooted in the understanding that all aspects of an individual's life are interconnected, and an imbalance in one area can affect the others. Rather than merely treating symptoms, holistic health seeks to address the root causes of health issues and promote long-term wellness.

The term "holistic" itself is derived from the Greek word "holos," meaning "whole" or "entire." Holistic health practitioners view each person as a unique individual, considering their lifestyle, environment, and personal history. This comprehensive perspective allows for personalized treatment plans that cater to the specific needs of the individual.

Holistic health is more than just a buzzword; it is a philosophy of health and wellness that has been practiced for centuries across various cultures. At its core, holistic health emphasizes the interconnectedness of the body, mind, and spirit, recognizing that true health is more than the absence of disease. It involves a harmonious balance of all aspects of our being. This chapter will introduce the fundamental concepts of holistic health, exploring its history, principles, and the benefits it offers.

The Origins and Evolution of Holistic Health

Holistic health practices have ancient roots, dating back thousands of years. In ancient India, the practice of Ayurveda emerged as a comprehensive system of medicine, focusing on balancing the body's energies, or doshas, through diet, herbs, and lifestyle changes. Traditional Chinese Medicine (TCM), another ancient system, uses acupuncture, herbal medicine, and Tai Chi to balance the body's vital energy, or Qi.

In the Western world, holistic health gained prominence in the 19th and 20th centuries, as practitioners began to seek alternatives to the reductionist approach of conventional medicine. This shift was fueled by a growing recognition of the limitations of treating symptoms without addressing underlying causes. Today, holistic health is embraced by a diverse range of practitioners and individuals seeking a more balanced and integrative approach to wellness.

The Difference Between Holistic and Conventional Health

Holistic and conventional health approaches represent two distinct paradigms of healthcare, each with its unique principles, methods, and goals. Understanding the differences between these approaches can help individuals make informed decisions about their health and wellness.

Holistic Health

Whole-Person Approach

Holistic health considers the whole person, including their physical, mental, emotional, and spiritual well-being. It emphasizes the interconnectedness of all aspects of health and seeks to address the root causes of health issues rather than just treating symptoms.

Preventive Focus

Holistic health places a strong emphasis on preventive care. It encourages lifestyle practices that promote overall wellness, such as balanced nutrition, regular exercise, stress management, and adequate sleep. The goal is to maintain health and prevent the onset of disease.

Personalized Care

Holistic health recognizes that each individual is unique and requires personalized treatment plans. Practitioners consider the patient's lifestyle, environment, and personal history to tailor treatments that meet their specific needs.

Integration of Therapies

Holistic health incorporates a wide range of therapies, blending conventional medical treatments with complementary and alternative practices. This may include acupuncture, herbal medicine, chiropractic care, yoga, meditation, and more.

Patient Empowerment and Education

Holistic health emphasizes educating and empowering individuals to take an active role in their health. Patients are encouraged to make informed choices and adopt self-care practices that support their well-being.

Conventional Health

Symptom and Disease Focus

Conventional health, often referred to as Western or allopathic medicine, focuses primarily on diagnosing and treating specific symptoms and diseases. It uses a scientific approach to identify and manage medical conditions, often through pharmaceuticals, surgery, and other medical interventions.

Reactive Approach

Conventional health tends to be more reactive, addressing health issues as they arise. While preventive measures like vaccinations and screenings are part of conventional medicine, the primary focus is on treating existing conditions.

Standardized Treatment

Conventional health often relies on standardized treatment protocols based on clinical guidelines and evidence-based practices. Treatments are generally uniform and follow established medical standards.

Specialized Care

Conventional health involves a high degree of specialization, with healthcare providers focusing on specific areas of medicine, such as cardiology, oncology, or neurology. This allows for targeted and advanced treatments for complex conditions.

5. Emphasis on Technology and Pharmaceuticals

Conventional health heavily utilizes advanced medical technology and pharmaceuticals to diagnose and treat conditions. Innovations in medical imaging, surgical techniques, and drug development are central to conventional medical practice.

Key Differences

Approach to Health

Holistic Health: Focuses on the whole person, addressing physical, mental, emotional, and spiritual aspects.

Conventional Health: Focuses on specific symptoms and diseases, often using a reductionist approach.

The Multifaceted Benefits of Holistic Health

Holistic health, a philosophy and practice that considers the whole person, including their physical, mental, emotional, and spiritual well-being, offers a comprehensive approach to achieving optimal health. Unlike conventional medicine, which often focuses on treating symptoms, holistic health aims to address the root causes of health issues and promote overall balance. The benefits of this integrative approach are profound and wide-ranging, encompassing preventive care, personalized treatment plans, stress reduction, enhanced physical health, mental and emotional balance, improved healing and recovery, disease prevention, greater self-awareness, improved quality of life, and sustainable health practices.

Comprehensive Wellness

At the heart of holistic health is the concept of comprehensive wellness. This approach recognizes that true health is achieved when all aspects of a person's life are in harmony. By considering physical, mental, emotional, and spiritual dimensions, holistic health ensures that no part of an individual's well-being is neglected. This comprehensive approach leads to a more balanced and harmonious state of being, which is essential for overall wellness.

Preventive Care

One of the most significant advantages of holistic health is its emphasis on preventive care. By adopting lifestyle practices that support wellness, such as balanced nutrition, regular exercise, and effective stress management, individuals can prevent the onset of chronic diseases and health issues. This proactive approach not only enhances quality of life but also reduces the need for medical interventions, making it a cost-effective strategy for long-term health.

Personalized Health Plans

Holistic health acknowledges the uniqueness of each individual, tailoring care plans to address specific needs. This personalized approach ensures that treatments and wellness strategies are designed to fit the individual, enhancing their effectiveness and leading to better health outcomes. By focusing on the person rather than just the symptoms, holistic health practitioners can provide more precise and effective care.

Stress Reduction

Stress is a significant factor contributing to various health issues, including hypertension, anxiety, and depression. Holistic health practices, such as mindfulness, meditation, yoga, and deep breathing exercises, have been shown to significantly reduce stress levels. These techniques promote relaxation and improve mental clarity, contributing to overall well-being. By incorporating these practices into daily routines, individuals can better manage stress and its associated health risks.

Enhanced Physical Health

Holistic health promotes the adoption of healthy lifestyle habits, including nutritious eating, regular physical activity, and adequate rest. These habits are crucial for maintaining and improving physical health. For example, balanced nutrition provides the body with essential nutrients, regular exercise enhances cardiovascular function and strengthens muscles, and adequate rest allows for recovery and rejuvenation. Collectively, these practices lead to a stronger immune system and improved overall health.

Mental and Emotional Balance

Mental and emotional well-being are integral components of holistic health. Practices such as counseling, life coaching, and stress management techniques support mental and emotional health by addressing emotional and psychological needs. Achieving mental and emotional balance helps individuals develop resilience, improve emotional stability, and enhance overall mental wellness. This balance is essential for coping with life's challenges and maintaining a positive outlook.

Improved Healing and Recovery

By focusing on the whole person, holistic health practices can accelerate the healing process and improve recovery outcomes. Integrative therapies, such as acupuncture, chiropractic care, and herbal medicine, complement conventional treatments and provide a well-rounded approach to healing. These therapies support the body's natural healing processes, leading to faster and more complete recovery.

Disease Prevention

Preventing disease is a key objective of holistic health. Adopting holistic health practices can significantly reduce the risk of developing chronic diseases. Preventive measures, such as balanced nutrition, regular physical activity, and stress management, are crucial in maintaining long-term health and preventing conditions such as diabetes, heart disease, and obesity. By focusing on prevention, holistic health helps individuals maintain their health and well-being throughout their lives.

Greater Self-Awareness

Holistic health practices often lead to increased self-awareness and a deeper understanding of one's body, mind, and spirit. This heightened awareness helps individuals make informed choices about their health and lifestyle, fostering a sense of empowerment and control over their well-being. Self-awareness is crucial for recognizing and addressing health issues early, leading to better health outcomes.

Improved Quality of Life

Ultimately, the goal of holistic health is to enhance the overall quality of life. By addressing all aspects of health and promoting balance, individuals can experience greater satisfaction, joy, and fulfillment in their lives. This holistic approach not only improves physical health but also enriches mental, emotional, and spiritual well-being, leading to a more fulfilling and meaningful life.

Sustainable Health Practices

Holistic health encourages sustainable and long-term health practices rather than quick fixes. By integrating holistic principles into daily routines, individuals can maintain their health and wellness over the long term. This approach leads to lasting benefits and a healthier lifestyle, ensuring that individuals can enjoy the advantages of holistic health throughout their lives.

The benefits of holistic health are vast and far-reaching, encompassing all aspects of an individual's well-being. By adopting a holistic approach to health, individuals can achieve comprehensive wellness, prevent disease, reduce stress, and improve their quality of life. Holistic health empowers individuals to take charge of their health, leading to a balanced, harmonious, and fulfilling life. This integrative approach not only addresses immediate health concerns but also promotes long-term health and wellness, making it a valuable strategy for achieving optimal health

Core Principles

Whole-Person Care

Holistic health treats individuals as whole beings, acknowledging that physical health cannot be separated from mental, emotional, and spiritual well-being. This approach recognizes that all aspects of a person's life are interrelated, and optimal health can only be achieved when all are in balance.

Preventive Care and Wellness

A key focus of holistic health is prevention and promoting overall wellness rather than merely addressing illnesses. By encouraging healthy lifestyle choices, stress management, and regular health check-ups, holistic health aims to prevent health issues before they arise.

Natural Healing

Holistic health emphasizes the use of natural remedies and therapies to support the body's innate healing abilities. This includes dietary changes, herbal medicine, acupuncture, and other natural therapies that work in harmony with the body's processes.

Patient-Centered Care

In holistic health, patients are actively involved in their own care and decision-making processes. This collaborative relationship between practitioners and patients empowers individuals to take charge of their health and make informed choices.

Integration of Multiple Therapies

Holistic health combines different therapeutic approaches for comprehensive care. This may include conventional medicine, alternative therapies, and lifestyle changes, providing a broad spectrum of options to address all aspects of health.

The Mind-Body Connection

A fundamental concept in holistic health is the mind-body connection, which acknowledges that mental and emotional states can significantly impact physical health. This interconnection means that stress, anxiety, and negative emotions can manifest as physical symptoms, while physical health issues can affect mental well-being.

Practices that nurture the mind-body connection include mindfulness meditation, yoga, and stress management techniques. These practices help individuals develop greater awareness of their thoughts and emotions, leading to improved mental clarity, reduced stress, and enhanced overall health.

Mindfulness Meditation: This practice involves paying attention to the present moment without judgment. By cultivating a state of mindfulness, individuals can reduce stress, enhance emotional regulation, and improve mental clarity.

Yoga: Combining physical postures, breathing exercises, and meditation, yoga promotes physical flexibility, mental relaxation, and spiritual growth. It helps to balance the mind and body, fostering a sense of inner peace and well-being.

Stress Management: Techniques such as deep breathing, progressive muscle relaxation, and visualization can help individuals manage stress effectively. By reducing the harmful effects of stress, these practices contribute to better physical and mental health.

Nutrition and Diet

Nutrition plays a pivotal role in holistic health. A balanced diet, rich in whole foods such as fruits, vegetables, whole grains, and lean proteins, supports the body's natural healing processes and helps prevent disease. Holistic nutritionists consider not only the nutritional content of food but also its source, preparation, and how it affects the individual's body and mind.

Whole Foods: Foods that are minimally processed and close to their natural state provide essential nutrients and antioxidants that support overall health. These include fresh fruits and vegetables, whole grains, nuts, seeds, and lean proteins.

Hydration: Drinking adequate water is crucial for maintaining bodily functions, from digestion to temperature regulation. Proper hydration supports overall health and well-being.

Mindful Eating: Paying attention to how and what you eat can enhance digestion and nutrient absorption. Mindful eating involves savoring each bite, being aware of hunger and fullness cues, and appreciating the sensory experience of eating.

Physical Activity

Regular physical activity is essential for maintaining physical health, improving mood, and reducing the risk of chronic diseases. Holistic health encourages finding forms of exercise that you enjoy and that align with your lifestyle, promoting long-term adherence and overall well-being.

Aerobic Exercise: Activities like walking, running, and swimming boost cardiovascular health and improve stamina. Regular aerobic exercise can help maintain a healthy weight, reduce stress, and enhance overall fitness.

Strength Training: Building muscle through resistance exercises supports metabolic health, improves bone density, and enhances physical strength. Strength training can also help prevent injuries and improve functional abilities.

Flexibility and Balance: Practices like stretching, yoga, and tai chi improve flexibility and coordination, reducing the risk of injury. These exercises also promote relaxation and mental clarity, contributing to overall well-being.

Environmental Factors

The environment in which you live and work can significantly impact your health. Holistic health advocates for creating spaces that promote well-being and reduce exposure to toxins. This includes both the physical environment and the social environment, which can influence mental and emotional health.

Clean Living Spaces: Reducing clutter and ensuring good ventilation can enhance mental clarity and physical health. A clean and organized environment promotes relaxation and reduces stress.

Natural Products: Using natural cleaning and personal care products can minimize exposure to harmful chemicals. Choosing eco-friendly products supports both personal health and environmental sustainability.

Green Spaces: Spending time in nature has been shown to reduce stress, improve mood, and enhance overall well-being. Engaging with natural environments can foster a sense of peace and connection with the world around you.

Spiritual Health

Spiritual health, although often overlooked, is a vital component of holistic well-being. It involves finding meaning and purpose in life, which can provide a sense of peace and resilience. Spiritual health is deeply personal and can be nurtured through various practices and beliefs.

Spiritual Practices: Engaging in practices such as prayer, meditation, or attending religious services can nurture your spiritual health. These practices provide a sense of connection to something greater than oneself and offer comfort and guidance.

Community and Connection: Building and maintaining supportive relationships with family, friends, and community can enhance your sense of belonging and emotional support. Social connections are vital for mental and emotional health.

Purpose and Meaning: Reflecting on your values, goals, and what gives your life meaning can contribute to a deeper sense of fulfillment. Understanding your purpose can provide direction and motivation, enhancing overall well-being.

Holistic health is a comprehensive approach that recognizes the complexity of human well-being. By considering the whole person and addressing the interconnectedness of physical, mental, emotional, and spiritual dimensions, holistic health offers a path to a more balanced and fulfilling life. This chapter has explored the defining principles of holistic health, the importance of the mind-body connection, the role of nutrition and physical activity, the impact of environmental factors, and the significance of spiritual health.

As you continue to explore holistic health, remember that it is a dynamic and evolving journey. Embrace the principles and practices that resonate with you and be open to discovering new ways to enhance your overall well-being. By nurturing all aspects of your life, you can achieve a state of harmony and balance that supports your health and happiness.

The Importance of Balanced Nutrition in Holistic Health

Balanced nutrition is a cornerstone of holistic health, playing a critical role in maintaining overall well-being. In holistic health, which emphasizes the interconnectedness of the body, mind, and spirit, balanced nutrition serves as a fundamental building block that supports all aspects of an individual's health. This essay explores the importance of balanced nutrition in holistic health, highlighting its impact on physical, mental, emotional, and spiritual well-being.

Fueling the Body

Balanced nutrition is essential for maintaining physical health. The body requires a variety of nutrients to function optimally, and a well-rounded diet ensures that these needs are met. Key components of balanced nutrition include:

Macronutrients and Micronutrients

A balanced diet provides the necessary macronutrients—carbohydrates, proteins, and fats—that supply energy and support bodily functions. Carbohydrates are the body's primary energy source, proteins are crucial for tissue repair and growth, and fats are essential for hormone production and brain health. In addition to macronutrients, micronutrients such as vitamins and minerals are vital for various biochemical processes. For example, vitamin C supports the immune system, calcium strengthens bones, and iron is necessary for oxygen transport in the blood.

Immune System Support

Proper nutrition strengthens the immune system, making the body more resilient to infections and diseases. Nutrients like vitamin C, vitamin D, zinc, and antioxidants play critical roles in immune function. A diet rich in fruits, vegetables, whole grains, lean proteins, and healthy fats provides these essential nutrients, helping to keep the immune system robust and responsive.

Chronic Disease Prevention

Balanced nutrition is instrumental in preventing chronic diseases such as obesity, diabetes, cardiovascular disease, and certain cancers. Diets high in processed foods, sugars, and unhealthy fats are linked to an increased risk of these conditions. Conversely, diets rich in whole, unprocessed foods, including plenty of fruits, vegetables, whole grains, and lean proteins, are associated with a lower risk of chronic diseases. Maintaining a healthy weight through balanced nutrition also reduces the burden on the body's systems, further preventing disease.

Mental and Emotional Health: Nourishing the Mind

The connection between diet and mental health is well-established, with balanced nutrition playing a pivotal role in cognitive function and emotional stability.

Cognitive Function and Brain Health

The brain requires a constant supply of nutrients to function effectively. Omega-3 fatty acids, found in fish, flaxseeds, and walnuts, are crucial for brain health and cognitive function. These healthy fats support the structure of brain cells and enhance communication between neurons. Antioxidants, found in berries, leafy greens, and nuts, protect the brain from oxidative stress and inflammation, which can impair cognitive function. Additionally, B vitamins, particularly folate and B12, are essential for neural health and cognitive performance.

Emotional Stability

Diet influences neurotransmitter production, which affects mood and emotional well-being. For instance, the amino acid tryptophan, found in foods like turkey, eggs, and nuts, is a precursor to serotonin, a neurotransmitter that regulates mood and promotes feelings of well-being. Similarly, carbohydrates aid in the absorption of tryptophan, further supporting serotonin production. Diets high in refined sugars and processed foods, however, can lead to fluctuations in blood sugar levels, contributing to mood swings, anxiety, and depression. Consuming a balanced diet that includes complex carbohydrates, healthy fats, and proteins helps stabilize blood sugar levels and supports emotional health.

Spiritual Health: Fostering Connection and Mindfulness

In holistic health, spiritual well-being is recognized as an integral component of overall health. Balanced nutrition can enhance spiritual health by fostering a sense of connection, mindfulness, and gratitude.

Mindful Eating

Practicing mindful eating involves paying attention to the experience of eating, savoring each bite, and listening to the body's hunger and satiety cues. This practice encourages a deeper connection with food and an appreciation for its role in nourishing the body. Mindful eating can transform meals into opportunities for reflection and gratitude, enhancing spiritual well-being. It also helps individuals make healthier food choices, as they become more attuned to how different foods affect their bodies and minds.

Connection with Nature

Choosing whole, unprocessed foods that are locally sourced and sustainably grown can foster a sense of connection with nature. Understanding where food comes from and the effort involved in its production can inspire gratitude and respect for the environment. This connection can enhance spiritual health by promoting a sense of interconnectedness with the natural world and encouraging sustainable living practices.

Integrative Approach: Combining Nutrition with Other Holistic Practices

Balanced nutrition does not exist in isolation; it is most effective when integrated with other holistic health practices. Combining proper nutrition with regular exercise, adequate sleep, stress management techniques, and spiritual practices creates a comprehensive approach to health that addresses all dimensions of well-being.

Synergistic Effects

The synergistic effects of combining balanced nutrition with other holistic practices can amplify the benefits. For example, regular exercise enhances the body's ability to utilize nutrients effectively, while adequate sleep supports the metabolic processes involved in nutrient assimilation and energy production. Stress management techniques, such as meditation and yoga, can improve digestion and nutrient absorption by reducing the negative impact of stress on the gastrointestinal system. Together, these practices create a holistic lifestyle that supports optimal health and well-being.

Balanced nutrition is a fundamental pillar of holistic health, essential for maintaining physical, mental, emotional, and spiritual well-being. By providing the body with the necessary nutrients, balanced nutrition supports immune function, prevents chronic diseases, enhances cognitive function, stabilizes mood, and fosters a deeper connection with food and nature. When combined with other holistic practices, balanced nutrition creates a comprehensive approach to health that promotes harmony and balance in all aspects of life. Embracing balanced nutrition as part of a holistic health regimen can lead to a more fulfilling, vibrant, and meaningful existence.

The Importance of Getting Vitamins from Food Sources and Other Sources

Vitamins are essential micronutrients that the body needs in small amounts to function correctly. They play critical roles in various physiological processes, including metabolism, immunity, and cellular repair. While it is possible to obtain vitamins from supplements, getting them from food sources is generally more beneficial due to the presence of other essential nutrients and the natural synergy of food components. Here, we will discuss the importance of obtaining vitamins from food sources, explain the purpose and benefits of each vitamin, and highlight both natural food sources and other sources.

Fat-Soluble Vitamins

Vitamin A

Purpose and Benefits:

- Supports vision, particularly night vision

- Promotes healthy skin and mucous membranes

- Enhances immune function

- Aids in reproduction and cellular communication

Food Sources:

- Liver, fish oils, milk, eggs

- Orange and yellow vegetables (carrots, sweet potatoes)

- Dark leafy greens (spinach, kale)

Other Sources:

- Supplements (retinol, beta-carotene)

- Fortified foods (cereals, dairy products)

Vitamin D

Purpose and Benefits:

- Promotes calcium absorption for healthy bones and teeth

- Supports immune function

- Plays a role in muscle function and cardiovascular health

Food Sources:

- Fatty fish (salmon, mackerel, sardines)

- Egg yolks

- Fortified dairy and plant milk

- Mushrooms exposed to sunlight

Other Sources:

- Sunlight exposure (synthesized by the skin)

- Supplements (vitamin D2, D3)

Vitamin E

Purpose and Benefits:

- Acts as an antioxidant, protecting cells from damage

- Supports immune function

- Enhances skin health and repair

Food Sources:

- Nuts and seeds (almonds, sunflower seeds)

- Vegetable oils (wheat germ oil, sunflower oil)

- Green leafy vegetables (spinach, broccoli)

Other Sources:

- Supplements (tocopherol, tocotrienol)

- Fortified foods (cereals, juices)

Vitamin K

Purpose and Benefits:

- Essential for blood clotting

- Supports bone health by regulating calcium metabolism

Food Sources:

- Green leafy vegetables (kale, spinach, broccoli)

- Fermented foods (natto)

- Certain vegetable oils

Other Sources:

- Supplements (phylloquinone, menaquinone)

- Fortified foods (some dairy products)

Water-Soluble Vitamins

Vitamin C (Ascorbic Acid)

Purpose and Benefits:

- Acts as an antioxidant

- Supports the immune system

- Promotes collagen production for healthy skin, cartilage, and bones

- Enhances iron absorption from plant-based foods

Food Sources:

- Citrus fruits (oranges, lemons)

- Berries (strawberries, raspberries)

- Vegetables (bell peppers, broccoli, Brussels sprouts)

Other Sources:

- Supplements (ascorbic acid, sodium ascorbate)

- Fortified foods (juices, cereals)

Vitamin B1 (Thiamine)

Purpose and Benefits:

- Supports energy metabolism

- Essential for nerve function and muscle contraction

Food Sources:

- Whole grains (brown rice, whole wheat)

- Legumes (beans, lentils)

- Nuts and seeds (sunflower seeds, flaxseeds)

- Pork

Other Sources:

- Supplements (thiamine hydrochloride)

- Fortified foods (breads, cereals)

7. Vitamin B2 (Riboflavin)

Purpose and Benefits:

- Supports energy production

- Acts as an antioxidant

- Promotes skin and eye health

Food Sources:

- Dairy products (milk, yogurt)

- Eggs

- Green leafy vegetables (spinach, broccoli)

- Meat and fish

Other Sources:

- Supplements (riboflavin)

- Fortified foods (cereals, breads)

Vitamin B3 (Niacin)

Purpose and Benefits:

- Supports energy metabolism

- Helps maintain healthy skin

- Promotes digestive system health

Food Sources:

- Meat and poultry (chicken, turkey)

- Fish (tuna, salmon)

- Whole grains

- Legumes

Other Sources:

- Supplements (nicotinic acid, niacinamide)

- Fortified foods (cereals, bread)

Vitamin B5 (Pantothenic Acid)

Purpose and Benefits:

- Essential for synthesizing coenzyme A (CoA), critical for fatty acid metabolism

- Supports energy production

Food Sources:

- Meat (chicken, beef)

- Whole grains

- Vegetables (broccoli, sweet potatoes)

- Eggs

Other Sources:

- Supplements (calcium pantothenate)

- Fortified foods (cereals, beverages)

Vitamin B6 (Pyridoxine)

Purpose and Benefits:

- Involved in amino acid metabolism

- Supports neurotransmitter synthesis

- Essential for red blood cell production

Food Sources:

- Poultry (chicken, turkey)

- Fish (salmon, tuna)

- Potatoes and starchy vegetables

- Non-citrus fruits (bananas)

Other Sources:

- Supplements (pyridoxine hydrochloride)

- Fortified foods (cereals, energy bars)

Vitamin B7 (Biotin)

Purpose and Benefits:

- Supports carbohydrate, fat, and protein metabolism

- Promotes healthy skin, hair, and nails

Food Sources:

- Eggs (particularly yolks)

  - Nuts and seeds

    - Legumes

  - Whole grains

Other Sources:

- Supplements (biotin)

- Fortified foods (meal replacement bars, drinks)

Vitamin B9 (Folate/Folic Acid)

Purpose and Benefits:

- Crucial for DNA synthesis and cell division

- Supports fetal development during pregnancy

  - Promotes red blood cell formation

Food Sources:

- Leafy green vegetables (spinach, kale)

  - Legumes (beans, lentils)

  - Fruits (oranges, bananas)

    - Whole grains

Other Sources:

- Supplements (folic acid)

- Fortified foods (breads, cereals)

13. Vitamin B12 (Cobalamin)

Purpose and Benefits:

- Essential for red blood cell formation

- Supports nervous system health

- Involved in DNA synthesis

Food Sources:

- Animal products (meat, fish, poultry)

- Dairy products (milk, cheese)

- Eggs

Other Sources:

- Supplements (cyanocobalamin, methyl cobalamin)

- Fortified foods (plant-based milks, cereals)

The Synergy of Food Sources

While supplements can help address specific deficiencies, obtaining vitamins from food sources offers several advantages. Whole foods provide a complex matrix of nutrients, including fiber, antioxidants, and phytochemicals, which work synergistically to enhance health. For example, an orange provides not only vitamin C but also fiber, potassium, and a variety of beneficial plant compounds. This synergy can enhance the absorption and efficacy of vitamins, contributing to overall health more effectively than isolated supplements.

Balanced nutrition, achieved through a varied diet rich in whole foods, is fundamental to holistic health. Vitamins obtained from food sources support physical, mental, emotional, and spiritual well-being by providing essential nutrients in their most bioavailable and synergistic forms. While supplements can be useful in certain circumstances, prioritizing nutrient-dense foods ensures a comprehensive and natural approach to meeting the body's vitamin needs, ultimately promoting long-term health and wellness.

How to Eat a Balanced Meal

Eating a balanced meal is crucial for maintaining good health and providing your body with the necessary nutrients it needs to function optimally. A balanced meal typically includes a variety of foods from different food groups, ensuring you get a mix of macronutrients (carbohydrates, proteins, and fats) and micronutrients (vitamins and minerals). Here are some practical steps and tips to help you eat a balanced meal:

1. Include a Variety of Food Groups

A balanced meal should contain a mix of the following food groups:

- **Vegetables**: Aim to fill half of your plate with a variety of colorful vegetables. They are low in calories and high in essential nutrients and fiber.

- **Fruits**: Include a serving of fruit, either as part of the main dish or as a dessert. Fruits are rich in vitamins, minerals, and fiber.

- **Grains**: Choose whole grains such as brown rice, quinoa, whole wheat bread, or oats. Whole grains provide more fiber and nutrients compared to refined grains.

- **Proteins**: Incorporate a source of lean protein, such as poultry, fish, beans, lentils, tofu, eggs, or low-fat dairy. Proteins are essential for muscle repair and overall body function.

- **Dairy or Dairy Alternatives**: Include a serving of dairy or fortified dairy alternatives for calcium and vitamin D. Options include milk, yogurt, cheese, or plant-based milks like almond or soy milk.

2. Balance Macronutrients

Ensure that your meal contains an appropriate balance of carbohydrates, proteins, and fats:

- **Carbohydrates**: Provide energy for your body. Choose complex carbohydrates like whole grains, fruits, and vegetables, which also offer fiber and other nutrients.

- **Proteins**: Essential for building and repairing tissues. Include lean protein sources like chicken, fish, beans, nuts, and seeds.

- **Fats**: Necessary for various bodily functions, including hormone production and nutrient absorption. Opt for healthy fats found in avocados, nuts, seeds, and olive oil.

3. Portion Control

Pay attention to portion sizes to avoid overeating. Use the following guidelines to help with portion control:

- **Vegetables and Fruits**: Fill half of your plate with vegetables and fruits.

- **Grains and Proteins**: Allocate one-quarter of your plate to whole grains and one-quarter to protein sources.

- **Fats**: Include healthy fats in moderation, such as a small handful of nuts or a tablespoon of olive oil.

4. Add Variety and Color

Eating a variety of foods ensures you get a wide range of nutrients. Different colors in fruits and vegetables often indicate different types of nutrients and antioxidants. Aim to eat a "rainbow" of colors by including various fruits and vegetables in your meals.

5. Mindful Eating

Practice mindful eating by paying attention to your hunger and fullness cues. Eat slowly, savor each bite, and avoid distractions like watching TV or using your phone while eating. This helps you enjoy your meal more and can prevent overeating.

6. Hydration

Don't forget to include a source of hydration. Water is the best choice, but you can also include herbal teas or other non-sugary beverages. Avoid sugary drinks and limit your intake of caffeinated beverages.

Sample Balanced Meal Ideas

Breakfast:

- **Oatmeal**: Cooked with milk or a dairy alternative, topped with fresh berries, a sprinkle of nuts, and a drizzle of honey.

- **Scrambled Eggs**: With spinach, tomatoes, and a slice of whole-grain toast.

- **Smoothie**: Made with spinach, banana, frozen berries, Greek yogurt, and a tablespoon of chia seeds.

Lunch:

- **Salad**: Mixed greens with grilled chicken, cherry tomatoes, cucumber, avocado, and a dressing made from olive oil and lemon juice.

- **Whole-Grain Wrap**: Filled with hummus, shredded carrots, mixed greens, and lean turkey slices.

- **Quinoa Bowl**: With roasted vegetables, chickpeas, feta cheese, and a tahini dressing.

Dinner:

- **Grilled Salmon**: Served with a side of brown rice, steamed broccoli, and a mixed green salad with a vinaigrette dressing.

- **Stir-Fry**: Made with tofu or chicken, a variety of colorful vegetables, and served over brown rice or quinoa.

- **Whole-Grain Pasta**: Tossed with a tomato-based sauce, sautéed vegetables, and lean ground beef or turkey, topped with a sprinkle of Parmesan cheese.

Snacks:

- **Greek Yogurt**: With a handful of nuts and a drizzle of honey.

- **Apple Slices**: With almond butter.

- **Veggie Sticks**: Carrot, cucumber, and bell pepper slices with hummus.

Eating a balanced meal involves including a variety of foods from different food groups, balancing macronutrients, controlling portions, adding variety and color, practicing mindful eating, and staying hydrated. By following these guidelines, you can ensure that your meals

provide the necessary nutrients for optimal health and well-being. Incorporate these principles

into your daily routine to enjoy the benefits of a balanced and nutritious diet.

The Benefits of Exercising

Regular exercise is a fundamental component of a healthy lifestyle, offering a wide range of physical, mental, and emotional benefits. Incorporating physical activity into your daily routine can lead to significant improvements in overall well-being. Here are some key benefits of exercising:

1. Improved Physical Health

Cardiovascular Health: Regular aerobic exercise strengthens the heart and improves circulation, reducing the risk of cardiovascular diseases such as heart attack, stroke, and high blood pressure. Activities like walking, running, swimming, and cycling help maintain a healthy heart.

Weight Management: Exercise helps regulate body weight by burning calories and building muscle mass. It boosts metabolism and aids in weight loss or maintenance, reducing the risk of obesity-related conditions such as diabetes and metabolic syndrome.

Bone and Joint Health: Weight-bearing exercises such as walking, jogging, and resistance training enhance bone density, reducing the risk of osteoporosis and fractures. Exercise also strengthens muscles and joints, improving flexibility and reducing the risk of injury.

Muscle Strength and Endurance: Strength training exercises, including lifting weights and using resistance bands, increase muscle mass, strength, and endurance. This helps in daily activities, improves athletic performance, and supports metabolic health.

2. Enhanced Mental and Emotional Well-Being

Stress Reduction: Physical activity stimulates the production of endorphins, the body's natural mood elevators. Exercise reduces stress hormones like cortisol and adrenaline, promoting relaxation and reducing anxiety.

Improved Mood: Regular exercise is linked to improved mood and a reduction in symptoms of depression. Activities like running, cycling, and yoga have been shown to alleviate depressive symptoms and boost overall emotional health.

Better Sleep: Exercise helps regulate sleep patterns, promoting deeper and more restful sleep. Regular physical activity can help alleviate insomnia and other sleep disorders, leading to improved energy levels and daytime alertness.

Enhanced Cognitive Function: Exercise increases blood flow to the brain, supporting cognitive functions such as memory, attention, and problem-solving. It also promotes neuroplasticity, the brain's ability to adapt and change, which is beneficial for learning and mental agility.

3. Increased Energy Levels

Regular physical activity boosts energy levels by improving cardiovascular health and enhancing the efficiency of the cardiovascular system. This leads to better oxygen and nutrient delivery to tissues, increasing overall stamina and reducing feelings of fatigue.

4. Chronic Disease Prevention

Diabetes Management: Exercise helps regulate blood sugar levels by increasing insulin sensitivity. This is particularly beneficial for individuals with type 2 diabetes or those at risk of developing the condition.

Cancer Prevention: Regular physical activity is associated with a reduced risk of certain types of cancer, including breast, colon, and lung cancer. Exercise helps regulate hormones and reduces inflammation, contributing to cancer prevention.

Improved Immune Function: Moderate exercise boosts the immune system by promoting the circulation of immune cells, enhancing the body's ability to fend off infections and illnesses.

5. Enhanced Longevity

Engaging in regular physical activity is linked to increased life expectancy. Exercise reduces the risk of chronic diseases, supports mental health, and enhances overall quality of life, contributing to a longer and healthier life.

6. Social Benefits

Community Engagement: Participating in group exercise activities, such as sports teams, fitness classes, or walking groups, fosters a sense of community and social connection. This can lead to new friendships, increased motivation, and a sense of belonging.

Family Bonding: Exercising with family members, such as going for walks, bike rides, or playing sports together, strengthens family bonds and promotes a healthy lifestyle for all members.

7. Improved Self-Esteem and Confidence

Achieving fitness goals, whether it's running a certain distance, lifting heavier weights, or mastering a new yoga pose, boosts self-esteem and confidence. Exercise also promotes a positive body image and self-perception.

8. Better Mobility and Balance

Regular exercise improves flexibility, balance, and coordination, reducing the risk of falls and enhancing mobility. This is particularly important for older adults, helping them maintain independence and a higher quality of life.

The benefits of exercising extend far beyond physical health, encompassing mental, emotional, and social well-being. By incorporating regular physical activity into your daily routine, you can improve cardiovascular health, manage weight, enhance mental health, increase energy levels, prevent chronic diseases, and enjoy a longer, more fulfilling life. Whether it's through aerobic exercises, strength training, flexibility exercises, or engaging in sports and recreational activities, the key is to find activities you enjoy and make them a regular part of your life. The positive impact of exercise on overall health and well-being cannot be overstated, making it an essential component of a healthy lifestyle.

The Benefits of Meditation

Meditation, a practice with ancient roots, has become increasingly popular in modern times due to its profound impact on mental, emotional, and physical well-being. By fostering a state of focused attention and relaxation, meditation offers a range of benefits that enhance overall health and quality of life. Here are some key benefits of meditation:

1. Stress Reduction

One of the most well-known benefits of meditation is its ability to reduce stress. By promoting relaxation and reducing the production of stress hormones such as cortisol, meditation helps calm the mind and body. Techniques such as mindfulness meditation, deep breathing, and progressive muscle relaxation are particularly effective in alleviating stress.

2. Enhanced Emotional Health

Improved Mood: Regular meditation practice is associated with improved mood and emotional stability. It helps reduce symptoms of anxiety, depression, and negative thinking by promoting a more balanced and positive mindset.

Increased Self-Awareness: Meditation fosters self-awareness by encouraging individuals to observe their thoughts and emotions without judgment. This heightened self-awareness can lead to better emotional regulation and a deeper understanding of oneself.

3. Better Focus and Concentration

Meditation practices, such as mindfulness and focused-attention meditation, improve focus and concentration. By training the mind to stay present and avoid distractions, meditation enhances cognitive abilities and productivity. This benefit is particularly valuable in today's fast-paced, multitasking world.

4. Improved Sleep Quality

Meditation can significantly improve sleep quality by promoting relaxation and reducing insomnia. Practices such as guided meditation and body scan meditation help calm the mind and prepare the body for restful sleep. Improved sleep quality, in turn, enhances overall health and well-being.

5. Reduced Symptoms of Anxiety and Depression

Anxiety Reduction: Meditation techniques, especially mindfulness meditation, have been shown to reduce symptoms of anxiety. By helping individuals stay grounded in the present moment, meditation reduces worry and rumination, which are common in anxiety disorders.

Alleviation of Depression: Regular meditation practice can also alleviate symptoms of depression. It promotes positive thinking and emotional resilience, reducing the severity and frequency of depressive episodes.

6. Enhanced Physical Health

Lower Blood Pressure: Meditation can help lower blood pressure by promoting relaxation and reducing stress. This benefit is particularly important for individuals with hypertension, as it reduces the risk of cardiovascular diseases.

Pain Management: Meditation practices such as mindfulness-based stress reduction (MBSR) and guided imagery can help manage chronic pain. By altering the perception of pain and promoting relaxation, meditation provides a natural and effective way to cope with pain.

Improved Immune Function: Regular meditation practice is associated with improved immune function. By reducing stress and promoting overall well-being, meditation enhances the body's ability to fight off infections and illnesses.

7. Enhanced Self-Discipline and Willpower

Meditation strengthens self-discipline and willpower by training the mind to focus and resist distractions. This benefit can extend to various aspects of life, including healthier eating habits, regular exercise, and better management of addictive behaviors.

8. Better Relationships

Improved Empathy and Compassion: Meditation practices, such as loving-kindness meditation, cultivate empathy and compassion. By fostering a sense of connection and understanding, these practices enhance interpersonal relationships and promote prosocial behavior.

Reduced Reactivity: Meditation helps individuals respond to situations more calmly and thoughtfully, reducing impulsive reactions and conflicts. This improved emotional regulation leads to healthier and more harmonious relationships.

9. Greater Creativity and Problem-Solving

Meditation enhances creativity and problem-solving abilities by promoting a state of relaxed, open awareness. By quieting the mind and allowing space for new ideas to emerge, meditation fosters creative thinking and innovation.

10. Spiritual Growth and Connection

For many individuals, meditation is a spiritual practice that fosters a deeper sense of connection and purpose. By promoting inner peace and self-awareness, meditation can lead to spiritual growth and a greater sense of meaning in life.

Meditation offers a wide range of benefits that enhance mental, emotional, and physical well-being. From reducing stress and improving emotional health to enhancing focus, sleep quality, and overall physical health, the positive impacts of meditation are profound and far-reaching. Whether practiced for spiritual growth, self-awareness, or stress reduction, meditation is a valuable tool for achieving a balanced and fulfilling life. Incorporating regular meditation practice into your daily routine can lead to significant improvements in overall health and quality of life, making it an essential component of holistic wellness.

The Benefits of Yoga

Yoga, an ancient practice that originated in India, combines physical postures, breathing exercises, meditation, and ethical principles to promote overall well-being. Over the centuries, yoga has evolved and been embraced worldwide for its numerous health benefits, encompassing the physical, mental, and spiritual aspects of life. Here are some key benefits of practicing yoga:

1. Improved Physical Health

Flexibility: Regular yoga practice enhances flexibility by stretching muscles and joints. Postures such as forward bends, backbends, and twists help increase the range of motion and reduce stiffness.

Strength: Yoga strengthens muscles through various poses that require holding and balancing body weight. Asanas like plank pose, warrior poses, and chair pose build core, leg, and upper body strength.

Balance and Coordination: Yoga improves balance and coordination through poses that challenge stability, such as tree pose and eagle pose. Enhanced balance reduces the risk of falls and improves overall body control.

Cardiovascular Health: Certain styles of yoga, such as Vinyasa and Ashtanga, provide cardiovascular benefits by increasing heart rate and improving circulation. Regular practice can enhance cardiovascular endurance and promote heart health.

Respiratory Function: Pranayama, or yogic breathing exercises, enhance respiratory efficiency by strengthening the diaphragm and increasing lung capacity. Improved breathing techniques support overall respiratory health.

Weight Management: Yoga aids in weight management by promoting physical activity, mindfulness, and healthy lifestyle choices. Regular practice helps burn calories, build muscle, and improve metabolism.

2. Enhanced Mental Health

Stress Reduction: Yoga is renowned for its ability to reduce stress. The combination of physical movement, breath control, and meditation calms the nervous system and lowers cortisol levels, promoting relaxation.

Improved Mood: Regular yoga practice boosts mood by increasing levels of neurotransmitters like serotonin and dopamine. It also stimulates the production of endorphins, which are natural mood elevators.

Anxiety and Depression Relief: Yoga helps alleviate symptoms of anxiety and depression by promoting relaxation and reducing negative thought patterns. Practices such as restorative yoga and mindfulness meditation are particularly effective in managing mental health conditions.

Increased Self-Awareness: Yoga fosters self-awareness by encouraging mindfulness and introspection. This heightened awareness helps individuals understand their thoughts, emotions, and behaviors, leading to greater self-acceptance and personal growth.

3. Better Sleep Quality

Yoga improves sleep quality by promoting relaxation and reducing insomnia. Practices such as gentle yoga, yin yoga, and yoga nidra (yogic sleep) prepare the body and mind for restful sleep. Improved sleep quality enhances overall health and well-being.

4. Enhanced Emotional Well-Being

Emotional Balance: Yoga helps regulate emotions by reducing stress and promoting a sense of calm. Practices like breathwork and meditation improve emotional resilience and stability.

Compassion and Empathy: Yoga encourages compassion and empathy by promoting mindfulness and connection with others. Practices such as loving-kindness meditation (metta) cultivate a sense of empathy and kindness towards oneself and others.

5. Spiritual Growth and Connection

For many practitioners, yoga is a spiritual practice that fosters a deeper sense of connection and purpose. The practice encourages self-reflection, inner peace, and a sense of unity with the surrounding world. Spiritual growth through yoga can lead to a greater sense of meaning and fulfillment in life.

6. Improved Cognitive Function

Concentration and Focus: Yoga enhances concentration and focus by promoting mindfulness and mental clarity. Practices like meditation and balancing poses improve attention span and cognitive function.

Memory and Learning: Yoga supports brain health by increasing blood flow to the brain and promoting neuroplasticity. Regular practice can enhance memory, learning, and overall cognitive abilities.

7. Enhanced Immune Function

Yoga boosts immune function by reducing stress, promoting relaxation, and supporting overall health. Practices such as pranayama and meditation enhance the body's ability to fight off infections and illnesses.

8. Pain Management

Yoga helps manage chronic pain conditions by promoting physical activity, reducing stress, and improving mental health. Gentle yoga and restorative practices provide relief from conditions like arthritis, lower back pain, and migraines.

9. Increased Energy and Vitality

Regular yoga practice increases energy levels and vitality by improving physical fitness, reducing stress, and promoting relaxation. Practices such as sun salutations and breathwork invigorate the body and mind, enhancing overall energy levels.

10. Social Connection and Community

Practicing yoga in a group setting fosters a sense of community and social connection. Group classes and yoga workshops provide opportunities to meet like-minded individuals, share experiences, and build supportive relationships.

The benefits of yoga extend across physical, mental, emotional, and spiritual dimensions, making it a holistic practice that promotes overall well-being. From improving flexibility, strength, and cardiovascular health to reducing stress, enhancing mood, and fostering spiritual growth, yoga offers a comprehensive approach to achieving and maintaining a balanced and fulfilling life.

Incorporating regular yoga practice into your daily routine can lead to significant improvements in health and quality of life, making it an invaluable component of a holistic wellness regimen. Whether practiced for physical fitness, mental health, spiritual growth, or social connection, yoga provides a versatile and effective pathway to enhanced well-being.

The Benefits of Herbalism

Herbalism, also known as herbal medicine, is the practice of using plants and plant extracts for medicinal purposes. It is one of the oldest forms of healthcare, with traditions dating back thousands of years across various cultures. In modern times, herbalism remains a popular and effective approach to promoting health and treating ailments. Here are some key benefits of herbalism:

1. Natural Healing

Holistic Approach: Herbalism treats the body as a whole, addressing the root causes of health issues rather than just alleviating symptoms. This holistic approach promotes overall well-being and balance.

Synergy of Compounds: Plants contain a complex mix of compounds that work synergistically to enhance their healing properties. This natural synergy can be more effective and safer than isolated synthetic drugs.

2. Fewer Side Effects

Gentler on the Body: Herbal remedies are generally gentler on the body compared to pharmaceutical drugs. They are less likely to cause adverse side effects when used appropriately.

Natural Balance: Herbs support the body's natural balance and healing processes. They often work with the body to restore health rather than forcing a specific reaction, reducing the likelihood of side effects.

10. Hormonal Balance

Menstrual and Menopausal Support: Herbs like black cohosh, chasteberry, and dong quai can help balance hormones and alleviate symptoms associated with menstruation and menopause.

Reproductive Health: Herbal remedies can support reproductive health by regulating menstrual cycles, improving fertility, and reducing symptoms of hormonal imbalances.

11. Cardiovascular Health

Heart Health: Herbs like hawthorn, garlic, and ginkgo biloba support cardiovascular health by improving blood circulation, reducing blood pressure, and lowering cholesterol levels.

Anti-Clotting Properties: Some herbs, such as garlic and ginger, have natural blood-thinning properties that can help prevent blood clots and reduce the risk of heart attacks and strokes.

Herbalism offers a natural, holistic approach to health and wellness, with a wide range of benefits for physical, mental, and emotional well-being. By harnessing the healing properties of plants, herbalism provides gentle, effective, and accessible remedies for various health conditions. Whether used for chronic disease management, immune support, mental health, or overall wellness, herbal remedies offer a valuable complement to conventional medicine. Embracing herbalism can lead to a more balanced, harmonious, and natural way of maintaining health and well-being. However, it is important to consult with a qualified healthcare provider before starting any herbal treatment to ensure safety and effectiveness.

The Benefits of Essential Oils

Essential oils, derived from plants through processes like distillation and cold pressing, have been used for centuries for their therapeutic properties. These concentrated extracts capture the essence of the plant's fragrance and healing potential. Essential oils are widely used in aromatherapy, personal care products, and natural remedies. Here are some key benefits of essential oils:

1. Stress Reduction and Relaxation

Aromatherapy: Essential oils like lavender, chamomile, and bergamot are commonly used in aromatherapy to reduce stress and promote relaxation. Inhaling these scents can help calm the mind, lower cortisol levels, and alleviate anxiety.

Relaxation: Oils such as ylang-ylang and sandalwood can help create a relaxing atmosphere, making them ideal for use in diffusers, bath soaks, or massage oils to unwind after a stressful day.

2. Improved Sleep Quality

Sleep Aid: Essential oils like lavender, valerian, and cedarwood are known for their sedative properties. They can help improve sleep quality by promoting relaxation and reducing insomnia.

Bedtime Rituals: Using essential oils in a bedtime routine, such as applying a few drops to a pillow or using a diffuser in the bedroom, can create a calming environment conducive to restful sleep.

3. Enhanced Mood and Emotional Well-Being

Mood Enhancement: Citrus oils like orange, lemon, and grapefruit are uplifting and can help improve mood and energy levels. These oils are often used to combat feelings of sadness or lethargy.

Emotional Balance: Essential oils like frankincense, clary sage, and rose have grounding and balancing effects, helping to stabilize emotions and promote a sense of well-being.

4. Immune System Support

Antimicrobial Properties: Many essential oils, such as tea tree, eucalyptus, and oregano, have antimicrobial properties that can help protect against bacteria, viruses, and fungi. These oils can be used in cleaning products or diffused to purify the air.

Immune Boosters: Oils like frankincense and lemon are believed to support the immune system by promoting overall health and resilience.

5. Pain Relief and Anti-Inflammatory Effects

Pain Management: Essential oils such as peppermint, eucalyptus, and ginger can provide natural pain relief. When applied topically (diluted in a carrier oil), they can help alleviate headaches, muscle pain, and joint discomfort.

Anti-Inflammatory: Oils like turmeric, chamomile, and helichrysum have anti-inflammatory properties that can reduce inflammation and swelling, providing relief from conditions like arthritis and sprains.

6. Respiratory Health

Congestion Relief: Essential oils like eucalyptus, peppermint, and rosemary are known for their ability to clear respiratory passages and reduce congestion. These oils can be inhaled through steam or diffused to ease breathing difficulties.

Respiratory Support: Oils such as tea tree and thyme have antibacterial properties that can help fight respiratory infections and support overall lung health.

7. Skin Care and Healing

Skin Health: Essential oils like tea tree, lavender, and geranium are beneficial for skin care. They can help treat acne, reduce inflammation, and promote healing of cuts and burns.

Anti-Aging: Oils such as frankincense and rosehip are rich in antioxidants and can help reduce the appearance of wrinkles, fine lines, and age spots, promoting youthful, healthy skin.

8. Digestive Health

Digestive Aid: Essential oils like peppermint, ginger, and fennel can aid digestion and alleviate symptoms such as bloating, indigestion, and nausea. These oils can be applied topically (diluted) or inhaled to support digestive health.

Stomach Comfort: Oils like chamomile and cardamom can help soothe the stomach and relieve digestive discomfort.

9. Cognitive Function and Focus

Mental Clarity: Essential oils like rosemary, basil, and peppermint are known for their ability to enhance cognitive function, improve concentration, and boost memory. These oils are beneficial for studying, working, or any activity requiring mental focus.

Alertness: Citrus oils such as lemon and orange can help increase alertness and reduce mental fatigue, making them useful for combating sluggishness and improving productivity.

10. Natural Cleaning and Household Uses

Natural Disinfectant: Essential oils like tea tree, lemon, and eucalyptus have natural disinfectant properties and can be used in homemade cleaning products to keep the home clean and free from harmful microbes.

Air Purification: Diffusing essential oils like lavender, lemon, and tea tree can help purify the air, remove odors, and create a pleasant and healthy environment.

Essential oils offer a wide range of benefits that enhance physical, mental, and emotional well-being. From reducing stress and improving sleep to boosting the immune system and supporting skin health, these natural extracts provide a versatile and holistic approach to health and wellness. Incorporating essential oils into daily routines through aromatherapy, topical application, or household uses can lead to significant improvements in overall quality of life. However, it is important to use essential oils safely, diluting them properly and consulting with a healthcare professional, when necessary, especially for individuals with pre-existing conditions or those who are pregnant or breastfeeding.

The Benefits of Energy Healing

Energy healing is a holistic practice that involves manipulating the body's energy fields to promote physical, mental, and emotional well-being. Various forms of energy healing, such as Reiki, acupuncture, Qigong, and therapeutic touch, are based on the belief that a balanced flow of energy (or life force) is essential for health. Here are some key benefits of energy healing:

1. Stress Reduction and Relaxation

Calmness and Peace: Energy healing techniques, such as Reiki and therapeutic touch, induce a state of deep relaxation, promoting calmness and peace. This relaxation response can help lower stress hormones like cortisol, reducing overall stress levels.

Enhanced Relaxation: By promoting relaxation, energy healing helps to calm the mind and body, making it easier to manage stress and anxiety. This can lead to improved mental clarity and emotional balance.

2. Improved Emotional Health

Emotional Release: Energy healing can help release trapped emotions and negative energy that contribute to emotional distress. Techniques like Reiki and emotional freedom techniques (EFT) facilitate emotional release, leading to improved mood and emotional stability.

Emotional Balance: Energy healing promotes emotional balance by harmonizing the body's energy fields. This can help reduce symptoms of anxiety, depression, and emotional turbulence.

3. Enhanced Physical Health

Pain Relief: Many forms of energy healing, such as acupuncture and Qigong, are effective in managing chronic pain. By balancing the body's energy, these practices can reduce pain and inflammation, promoting overall physical health.

Accelerated Healing: Energy healing can accelerate the body's natural healing processes by enhancing energy flow to affected areas. This can support recovery from injuries, surgeries, and illnesses.

Boosted Immune System: By promoting relaxation and reducing stress, energy healing can strengthen the immune system. A balanced energy system supports the body's ability to fight off infections and illnesses.

4. Improved Sleep Quality

Better Sleep: Energy healing can improve sleep quality by promoting relaxation and reducing insomnia. Techniques like Reiki and acupressure help calm the nervous system, making it easier to fall asleep and stay asleep.

Sleep Disorders: By addressing underlying energy imbalances, energy healing can help alleviate sleep disorders, leading to more restorative sleep and enhanced overall well-being.

5. Mental Clarity and Focus

Enhanced Concentration: Energy healing practices can clear mental fog and improve focus. By balancing the energy fields, techniques like Reiki and Qigong enhance mental clarity and cognitive function.

Reduced Mental Fatigue: Energy healing helps reduce mental fatigue by promoting relaxation and restoring energy levels. This can lead to improved productivity and mental performance.

6. Spiritual Growth and Connection

Deepened Spiritual Awareness: Energy healing can deepen spiritual awareness and connection. Practices like Reiki and Qigong promote a sense of inner peace and connection with the universe, enhancing spiritual growth.

Intuition and Insight: By balancing the body's energy, energy healing can enhance intuition and insight. This heightened awareness can lead to greater self-understanding and personal growth.

7. Holistic Healing

Whole-Person Healing: Energy healing addresses the whole person, including the physical, mental, emotional, and spiritual aspects of health. This holistic approach promotes overall well-being and harmony.

Integration with Other Therapies: Energy healing can be integrated with other therapeutic modalities, such as conventional medicine, psychotherapy, and physical therapy, to enhance overall health and healing outcomes.

8. Increased Energy and Vitality

Boosted Energy Levels: Energy healing can boost energy levels by clearing energy blockages and promoting a balanced flow of energy throughout the body. This can lead to increased vitality and a greater sense of well-being.

Vitality and Wellness: Regular energy healing sessions can help maintain balanced energy, promoting sustained vitality and wellness.

9. Improved Relationships

Emotional Healing: By promoting emotional balance and release, energy healing can improve interpersonal relationships. Reduced emotional reactivity and enhanced emotional stability contribute to healthier and more harmonious relationships.

Empathy and Compassion: Energy healing can enhance empathy and compassion by fostering a deeper connection with oneself and others. This can lead to improved communication and stronger emotional bonds.

10. Personal Empowerment and Growth

Self-Empowerment: Energy healing promotes self-empowerment by encouraging individuals to take an active role in their healing journey. By becoming more attuned to their own energy, individuals can make informed choices about their health and well-being.

Personal Transformation: Energy healing can facilitate personal transformation by promoting self-awareness and spiritual growth. This can lead to profound changes in one's life, fostering a greater sense of purpose and fulfillment.

Energy healing offers a wide range of benefits that enhance physical, mental, emotional, and spiritual well-being. From reducing stress and improving sleep to promoting physical healing and spiritual growth, energy healing provides a holistic approach to achieving and maintaining optimal health. By balancing the body's energy fields, energy healing supports the body's natural ability to heal and promotes overall harmony and wellness. Whether used as a complementary therapy or a primary healing modality, energy healing can lead to significant improvements in overall quality of life, making it a valuable tool for holistic health and well-being.

Conclusion: Embracing the Path to Holistic Health

Holistic health approaches offer a comprehensive and integrative pathway to achieving and maintaining optimal well-being. By addressing the interconnected dimensions of physical, mental, emotional, and spiritual health, holistic practices foster balance and harmony in all aspects of life. This journey towards holistic health is not just about treating symptoms but understanding and nurturing the whole person, promoting a state of wellness that is sustainable and enriching. One of the most compelling aspects of holistic health is its recognition of the interconnectedness of various health dimensions. Physical health is intricately linked to mental and emotional well-being, and spiritual health provides a foundation for inner peace and resilience. By acknowledging and addressing these connections, holistic health practices ensure that all facets of an individual's life are nurtured and balanced. Holistic health emphasizes the importance of prevention and proactive wellness. Through balanced nutrition, regular physical activity, stress management, and mindfulness practices, individuals can prevent many common health issues and promote long-term health. This preventive approach not only enhances the quality of life but also reduces the need for medical interventions, contributing to a more sustainable and cost-effective healthcare system.

The personalized nature of holistic health care is another key benefit. Recognizing that each person is unique, holistic practitioners tailor their recommendations and treatments to meet individual needs and circumstances. This personalized approach ensures that healthcare is both effective and compassionate, addressing the specific challenges and goals of each person.

Holistic health does not reject conventional medicine; rather, it seeks to integrate it with complementary and alternative therapies to provide the best possible outcomes. This integrative approach allows for the use of a wide range of treatments and practices, ensuring that individuals have access to the most appropriate and effective care for their needs. By combining the strengths of different health disciplines, holistic health provides a more comprehensive and effective approach to wellness.

A significant aspect of holistic health is the empowerment and education of individuals. By providing the knowledge and tools needed to make informed health choices, holistic health practices encourage individuals to take an active role in their wellness journey. This empowerment leads to greater self-awareness, self-care, and ultimately, a higher quality of life.

Holistic health approaches also foster spiritual and emotional growth. Practices such as meditation, yoga, and energy healing promote inner peace, self-awareness, and emotional resilience. This spiritual and emotional well-being is a cornerstone of holistic health, providing a foundation for overall wellness and a fulfilling life.

Holistic health often involves a sense of community and connection. Whether through group yoga classes, meditation groups, or community-supported agriculture, these practices foster a sense of belonging and support. This communal aspect of holistic health enhances social well-being and creates a network of support for individuals on their wellness journey.

Embracing holistic health is a lifelong journey that requires commitment, self-awareness, and a willingness to explore various practices and disciplines. The rewards of this journey are profound, offering enhanced well-being, deeper connections with oneself and others, and a more balanced and fulfilling life.

By integrating the principles and practices of holistic health into your daily life, you can create a foundation for lasting wellness and personal growth. Whether you are just beginning your journey or have been practicing holistic health for years, the principles outlined in this book provide a roadmap for achieving and maintaining optimal health.

Holistic health is more than a set of practices; it is a way of life that embraces the whole person. It invites you to take an active role in your health, to seek balance and harmony, and to nurture your body, mind, and spirit. As you continue on your holistic health journey, remember that every step you take brings you closer to a state of true wellness. Embrace this journey with an open heart and mind, and enjoy the profound benefits that holistic health has to offer.

NOTES

Dedication

To all the seekers of wellness and balance,

This book is dedicated to those who strive to live a life of harmony and well-being, embracing the holistic journey of nurturing the mind, body, and spirit.

To my daughter and husband, whose love, patience, and encouragement make every step of this journey meaningful and rewarding. You are my daily reminders of the beauty of holistic living.

To my family, for their unwavering support and love, which has been the foundation of my journey in holistic health.

To my mentors and teachers, whose wisdom and guidance have illuminated the path to understanding the profound interconnectedness of all aspects of health.

To my friends, whose encouragement, support, and shared experiences have been a constant source of strength and joy.

To my clients and readers, for their trust and commitment to exploring the holistic path to wellness. Your stories and experiences continue to inspire and drive my passion for holistic health.

May this book serve as a source of knowledge, inspiration, and empowerment for all who seek to achieve a balanced and fulfilling life through holistic health.